Table of Contents

Intermittent Fasting For Women: The Ultimate Intermittent Fasting Beginner's Weight Loss Guide

By Brittany Samons

Introduction

Have you heard about intermittent fasting? What is it about and why more and more people are changing their eating habits? Intermittent fasting (known as IF) is not exactly a diet like Paleo Diet or The Zone Diet, it is more a lifestyle, a new way of eating in which the main purpose it's to get the most of your meals in less hours. It is about changing your eating schedule while losing weight.

Women are always in search of diets that help them become leaner, intermittent fasting could be a good option to get lean without starving. With intermittent fasting people can consume bigger meals in a shorter time period. Intermitting fasting is an easy method to lose bad fat and it is also a significant one. It seems to be a today's trend but this weight loss method has been out there for many years now.

Chapter 1. How Do You Start Intermittent Fasting?

The human body works in two different states; the fed state and the fasted state, we need to understand the difference between them before we start intermittent fasting. When our body is digesting and absorbing food it's said it remains in a fed state. This begins when we start eating and continues for five hours approximately while the body is digesting and absorbing the food we ate. In this state insulin levels are high and it will be difficult for the body to burn fat. We never consume the sugar stored in our body because we eat three to five meals a day, then our body will burn first sugar leaving apart the ability of using fat as fuel.

After five hours the body stops absorbing food. This is called post-absorptive state; it lasts from eight to twelve hours from your last meal (if your last meal was at 6:00 p.m. the post-absorptive state lasts until 6:00 a.m. approximately). Here is when the fasted state begins; our body will burn fat easier because now insulin levels are lower. So let's have this clear in the fed state you cannot burn fat, just in the fasted state, then the idea is to put our body into that state. Our bodies rarely get in the fasted state because it takes twelve hours from the last meal and we continue eating before it can begins, then while being in that fat burning state it doesn't matter how much food people eat or how often they exercise, what matters is changing the meals schedule, there is where intermittent fasting enters to the equation.

One of the best things about intermittent fasting is that it allows you to eat your favorite foods while continuing losing weight. With intermittent fasting it's easier for people to trust their hunger signals, they can eat because they are hungry not because they are bored or stressed.

Chapter 2. Give it a Try!

Consider giving intermittent fasting a try, there are some different ways to incorporate it into your lifestyle. It can be daily, weekly or alternating days. The ideal thing is to incorporate it gradually, by the way we have been fasting every day, yes you heard right, while we are sleeping we are in a fasting period, bet you haven't thought about it. Below there are five different intermittent fasting methods; each one of them will increase the time span of fasting.

a) Weekly Intermittent Fasting I think if you are just getting start with intermittent fasting, the best way to do it is once per week at first. Maybe you won't cut down all those calories but it will help you to get use to it and you will get the benefits of fasting for twenty-four hours. The greatest benefit of doing a 24-hour fast is breaking the mental barrier of fasting; completing a successful first round will help you realize you actually can survive without eat for some hours! Eat normal one day (2000 calories) and the next one eat less (500 calorie) and repeat it again. For the first two weeks you can have a healthy snack that helps you with the nutrients ingest your body needs. By the third week just eat the 500 calories on the fasting days. Do not workout on "down days", first you need to get used to it.

b) Alternate Day Fasting. This could be the second option once you have accomplished a 24-hour fasting and are getting used to it, now you can try an alternate day fasting. Here you can eat all day and then do a 24-hour fasting. This way you will go for longer periods before taking the next step. The idea is to stop eating for 24 hours once or twice a week it is allow to drink calorie free beverages at the end of the 24-hour period you can eat normally again. This way you will reduce your calories intake without limiting what you eat. Exercise is important to succeed too. Take it one step at the time, try to go without food for a certain timespan then increase it gradually while your body adjusts to the fasting phase. Experts suggest beginning the fasting in a busy day so you won't have to be worried about eating all time. A good thing is there are no restrictions about food either counting calories of course you are not going to eat a whole pizza!

c) Daily Intermittent Fasting (The Leangains Diet) Here you will follow the Leangains model, which consist in a 14-hour fast (for women) followed by an eight-hour eating period. You choose the schedules best suit you; you decide if you eat breakfast and a lunch (more like a big meal) or it could be lunch and dinner. You can have just a glass of water in the morning and then a few hours later get lunch. During the fasting period you won't consume calories, calorie-free sweeteners and diet soda is allowed as black coffee. Doing daily intermittent fasting allows women to get used to it easily and make it a daily habit, just need to learn eating at certain times. It would be easily if they do the fasting periods from night through mornings. By daily intermittent fasting you will have to eat bigger meals to get the same number of calories during the week, because you are cutting a meal from your schedule. We don't mean that you have to be restrictive with your schedules on a 100%, if you have a late dinner or a breakfast with your friends you can eat at that time. Remember it is a lifestyle not a starving diet. Foods to eat will depend on the exercise you do, if you exercise is important to eat carbs and protein consumption should be regular and choose fresh food over processed foods. A protein shake it's also accepted if you are exercising a lot.

d) The fasting phase of The Warrior Diet The purpose of this is to fast about twenty hours a day and to eat just a large meal at night. The key is feeding the body with the nutrients it needs. People who adopt this method are programmed for eating at nights. Okay it sounds worse than it is: during the twenty hour fast you will be able to eat raw vegetables, fruit and a few servings of protein. This will help your body to boost energy and at the same time will stimulate fat burning. The objective of eating at night is to let the body recuperate, relax and consume the necessary nutrients. Here the fat burning will take place during the day. No too much carbohydrate is recommended with this method. Many people like it this way because they can still eat small snacks during the fasting period and that makes it easier to get through. People report fat loss and higher energy levels.

e) All combined (Fat Loss Forever) This method takes the best of all the methods we have mention above and combines it into one plan. This is about going on a 36-hour fast (okay this is not for everyone). Experts suggest going on the longest fasts for your busiest days and trying to avoid focusing on hunger. They also suggest exercising. Fat Loss Forever is based on a seven-day schedule for fasting and one cheat day.

These methods mention above are the "most popular" or well known in how to intermittent fasting but there are many others. Of course it is important to know that if you have a medical condition or a chronic disease it's better to consult your doctor before trying intermittent fasting. For women it would be a little bit harder than for men to fasting because of hormones issues so begin with a short fasting period and increase it gradually. At first it would be challenging but everything it's possible.

Of all the schedules mention above women have reported that the easiest practice is to skip breakfast, if you have your last meal at 6 p.m. and then eat your next meal next day at 12 p.m. you have fasted for 18 hours, enough time for your body to burn fat. You can drink a cup of black coffee or green tea in the morning will help you to feel satisfied until you next meal.

Chapter 3. Some Good Tips to Start Fasting

1) Set an objective. Thinking about what you want to achieve is a good way to start intermittent fasting. Goals can vary, it can be losing body fat or extending lifetime, increasing body mass, whatever it is thinking about it will motivate you. Just remember to set smart goals that you can achieve one by one. The first one could be loss fat then it could be tone your body, get a healthy lifestyle, etc.

2) Take your time. If you are decided to intermittent fasting keep it to your own pace, maybe first arrange your meals schedule, then go fasting for eight hours and continue with it gradually. If you go for a long term intermittent fasting for the first time probably you will feel exhausted with headaches. There is no rush right.

3) Don't pay attention to everything you hear. Don't listen to rumors, people talk without knowledge, your metabolism won't get slow, you won't lose muscle. Instead of listening here and there get informed, research, read articles about IF. Then make your decision about going fastening.

4) Grab a bottle of water. It will be much easier to get through the fasting periods if you drink plenty of water each time you focus on hunger. Instead of eating something between meals drink water, if it is your first time intermittent fasting you can drink some unsweetened drinks maybe tea or black coffee. This will make you fill full without adding extra pounds.

5) No more cravings. No more processed foods, if you are eating less time healthy food is the best choice. Goodbye sodas, cereal, candies, brownies, muffins and hello fresh fruits and vegetables. Remember no more visits to the vending machine.

6) Eat exactly the same way. When you finish your fasting period eat the same kind of meal you were used to eat before starting IF. You are not supposed to restrict meals size just hours. It is important to not restrict your meals size.

7) Sleep and fast at the same time. At least you will be sleeping for eight hours and there will be just six more hours in the morning that you can spend taking a bath, reading the morning newspaper, driving to work. Fast overnight!

8) Think about it like a good thing. Avoid thinking you are going on a diet and that you will be starving; think about it like your new lifestyle, like something good is happening to your body. If you keep bad thoughts about "dieting" or "fasting" and look at it as a torture it's probably you won't achieve your goals.

9) Busy Bee. Don't forget to start with intermittent fasting on a busy day when you won't be thinking to eat every two hours. Don't start it on a lazy Sunday! The whole idea is to being busy through the day so you don't have time to think about food. When people get bored cravings appear and you don't want to fail at your first try.

10) Move that body. You will get better results if you combine intermittent fasting with exercise. Nothing too heavy just move your body two or three days a week. If you are no such a sporty person you can start with a 30-minute walk every two days. Walking your dog everyday around the block could help too!

11) Be Patient. Cutting down calories and carbohydrates will bring results but it will take some time (al least two weeks), so be persistent and patient meanwhile grab a healthy snack! If you have enough patience and choose the right foods to eat your body as well as your brain will adapt in a short time.

12) Listen to your body. You are the one that knows your body better, be aware of signals, how do you feel while fasting, notice if they are significant changes in your appetite, your sleep, your energy levels and how you look. If you are not sure you can first pay a visit to your doctor.

13) Look around. It is not just about intermittent fasting, it also involves your environment, how many stress do you have, how long does it take you to recover from exercise, how well is fasting fitting in your life. Remember to eat well, healthy and fresh foods, sleep at least eight hours every night, laugh, go out with your friends and be happy.

Eat whole foods is better to start intermittent fasting it would be easier if you already eat clean (no processed foods) or when you follow a low carb diet. Women who have tried these before report to easily jump into intermittent fasting. If you are struggling with IF try first to get healthier eating habits, this way your body will adapt faster to fasting.

Now that you have a general idea of what is intermittent fasting let's talk about benefits. Intermittent fasting brings lots of benefits with it regarding to what some people say, you can lose weight and still get more benefits.

Chapter 4. Intermittent Fasting Benefits

Women are intended to try intermittent fasting for its loss weight results but it brings more benefits than they realize.

1) Keeps your sugar in place Sugar is known for being a source of energy for the body but it's not as good as it sounds, if we consume it in big amounts in processed foods it will promote insulin resistance this one is a driver of chronic diseases like cancer. With intermittent fasting the body gets used to burn fat instead of sugar as a primary fuel, then reduces the risk of diseases. Cancer cells use sugar to flourish; they cannot use fat!

2) No oxidation Fasting helps by reducing the accumulation of oxidative radicals in cells prevents aging and diseases.

3) Detox Our body is used to detox and cleanse, it is an automatic process for it but each time we get food we slow it down because the body focuses in digesting food. If we give our body fasting time it could focus on cleansing instead of processing that burger we ate.

4) Regulate Hormones (Pay attention ladies!) Intermittent fasting increases human growth hormone that helps the body repairing muscles and slows the aging process. Other hormones are leptin and ghrelin. Leptin regulates fat storage and tells the brain when fat levels are fine. Ghrelin is the one who sends hunger signs to the brain; these two will be normal with fasting cycles. Intermittent fasting and low sugar consumption will help the brain to pay attention when leptin hormone is saying enough.

5) Lose those extra pounds. If the body doesn't need sugars in a certain moment, sugars are stored as glycogen and when it reaches its maximum level then they are stored as fat. The glycogen is the first thing the body burns, by fasting you give time to your body to burn glycogen and then to continue with fat. So please let you body do its thing!

6) Back to the basics. With modern life comes processed foods, fast food, frozen food, we can find everything in a package these days. Guess what? An apple never tastes so good like when it's the first thing you eat after fasting. You will become more receptive to natural flavors, in fruits, vegetables and all fresh foods.

7) Makes you life way easier Eating three meals a day always take a significant time by preparing them. Intermittent fasting reduces the number of meals a day, this means less planning, less stress and more free time to do other activities.

8) Live a longer life. It is known that restricting calories will help to lengthening life, but it also means people are starving to get there. Who wants to spend the rest of its life restricting meals just to live a few more years? Intermittent fasting activates some mechanisms that work in the same way like if you were starving also you are not. A longer life without restricting calories!

9) Concentration. Observe people who eats a big breakfast is less focus and sleepy intermittent fasting will help you having more natural energy and being more focus. Your body won't be in a zombie state anymore!

10) No more dieting. Almost every time women come with a new diet they failed and they didn't get the desire results. One of the reasons is because they are eating the wrong foods, or because they don't follow it for a long term. Intermittent fasting is about changing eating behaviors and it is very easy to implement in your life and to adapt to it. One of the benefits of intermittent fasting is the sense of freedom from eating; enjoy eating when it feels right.

10) No more counting. Women spend so much time counting calories all because of diets, isn't that exhausting? Then why continue with this, your body doesn't worry about calories, if you exceed one day then fasting the next day, this way you can establish a balance. Stop worrying about calories.

A diet is easy on contemplation but when people really try to follow it, they quickly begin to miss eggs and meat and get bored of bananas and jelly. Then they failed trying to follow it. It is also more complicated because you need to prepare exclusively a certain meal for a certain day.

In the other hand intermittent fasting looks very hard in contemplation, people think they couldn't go without food for so many hours, but then once they start it, it's a total change in their lives.

Chapter 5. Low Calorie Recipes

It is very easy to prepare a lunch or dinner for a fasting day. Here there are some low calorie recipes for breakfast, lunch and dinner that are delicious and you can eat without starving.

Grilled Cheese Sandwich With Pear

279 Calories 4 Servings

Ingredients

- 8 loaves of bread (choose whole brain bread)

- 4 Cheddar cheese slices

- 2 fresh pears thinly sliced

- Spray oil

- Mayonnaise (optional)

Step 1 First preheat a large pan, medium heat.

Step 2 Place a cheddar cheese slice on a loaf of bread and two pear slices if you are using mayonnaise spread it on the bread. Place another loaf of bread on top. Spray a little oil on the pan.

Step 3 Place the sandwiches on the pan and grilled them for about 3 minutes turn once and wait until bread get slightly brown and crispy and cheese is melted.

This sandwich will be a delicious lunch and it takes about ten minutes to prepare it.

275 calories, 4 servings

Ingredients

- 4 fresh tilapia fillets

- 1 can (15 oz) of whole black beans, drained

- 1 can (10 oz) diced tomatoes, drained

- 1 cup of corn grains

- 1 small green onion, chopped

- 2 tablespoons of vegetable oil

- 1 tablespoon of cider vinegar

- 1/4 tablespoon of salt

Step 1 In a bowl toss the black beans, tomatoes, corn, chopped onion, vegetable oil and sprinkle in the vinegar. Set aside.

Step 2 Spray a skillet with oil and low heat. Sprinkle salt on top of the fillets; place them on the skillet and cook for about 3 minutes. Turn the fillets and cook for 2 more minutes or until the fish is well cooked.

Step 3 Serve a fillet on a plate with the bean and corn salad.

Quick Italian Chicken

237 calories, 4 servings

Ingredients

- 4 boneless and skinless chicken breasts

- 4 cups of broccoli florets (choose fresh broccoli instead of frozen)

- 1 can (14.5 oz) tomatoes, diced and drained

- 1/2 cup of italian dressing

Step 1 First preheat oven at 450°F. In a medium bowl mixed broccoli florets, tomatoes and dressing.

Step 2 For each package cut two foil rectangles (20 x 12 inches).

Step 3 Place a chicken breast on a foil rectangle, a spoonful of the vegetable mixed, cover with the other foil rectangle and wrap all to enclose.

Step 4 Place the packages in an oven tray. Cook for 25

minutes or until the chicken is not pink in the inside. Let the packages cool and carefully open them.

This is a super quickly and easy recipe perfect for a dinner.

Green, Red and Orange Salad

158 calories, 2 servings

Ingredients

- 1 can (10 oz) tomatoes, diced and drained

- 2 tablespoons of honey (natural not syrup)

- 1 tablespoon of rice vinegar

- 1 package (9 oz) of spinach (better is you used fresh spinach)

- 1 orange, peeled and chopped in little bits

- 1 avocado, peeled and diced

Step 1 First mixed the tomatoes, honey and vinegar in a small bowl.

Step 2 Add the spinach, the orange and the avocado to the mixed, toss and serve immediately.

Rice and Garden Vegetables

183 calories, 4 servings

Ingredients

- 1 tablespoon of butter (or margarine if you prefer)

- 3/4 cup of large grain rice, uncooked (choose brown rice)

- 1/2 teaspoon of garlic, minced

- 1-1/2 cup of low sodium chicken broth

- 1 cup of vegetables (choose your preferred)

- 1/8 teaspoon of salt

Step 1 Melt butter in a medium pan, medium heat. Add rice and garlic, cook for about 3 minutes or until garlic starts to smell, stirring often.

Step 2 Next add chicken broth and sprinkle salt to the pan, bring to boil. Cover the pan with a lid and low heat. Cook for about 20 minutes or until rice is tender.

Step 3 Serve as a side dish with chicken or steak.

As you can see these recipes are very fast and easy to prepare using healthy ingredients. So I suggest forgetting about all those restricting diets and embrace intermittent fasting. Enjoy your meal!

Conclusion

The first results you are going to observe is the way your body adapts to the new eating schedule. No more sugar and high carbs cravings but still eating until being full and satisfied, no more days of counting calories. Intermittent fasting will freed you from dieting and loss-regain cycle. Definitely you will have a new relationship with food and the reasons why you eat, intermittent fasting will lead you to a healthier life it is not just about your body it is also about being healthy in mind.

Remember you can eat all what you want but preferably choose healthy foods that will help you to keep a balance between fasting and eating. Eat healthy fats like olive and coconut oil, nuts, butter, avocados and eggs; eat lean meats and fresh vegetables and fruits. You can research for easy low calorie recipes or why not buy a new cooking book, exercise, open your mind and discover intermittent fasting lifestyle.

I want to personally thank you for reading my book. I hope you found information in this book useful and I would be very grateful if you could leave your honest review about this book. I certainly want to thank you in advance for doing this.

9 781633 831377

Intermittent Fasting For Women:

The Ultimate Intermittent Fasting Beginner's Weight Loss Guide

By

Brittany Samons